# AI Brain Healing & Stroke Recovery

How Smart Algorithms Help the Brain Repair Itself

*By Joe Correa*

Published by Live Stronger Faster



This book is for educational and informational purposes only. The author and publisher are not engaged in rendering legal, financial, or other professional advice. Readers should consult a qualified professional before making any financial decisions.

First Edition

# Table of Contents

# Introduction

For most of modern history, damage to the human brain was considered permanent. A stroke, traumatic brain injury, or neurological event often marked a clear dividing line between "before" and "after"—a moment after which recovery was expected to be partial at best, and decline at worst. Patients were taught to accept limitations, families were told to prepare for lifelong care, and rehabilitation focused more on compensation than restoration. Yet quietly, over the past two decades, neuroscience has rewritten this narrative. The brain is not fixed. It is not static. It is not finished. It is adaptive, dynamic, and capable of remarkable repair under the right conditions. This understanding of neuroplasticity laid the foundation for a new era of brain healing—one now being accelerated at an unprecedented pace by artificial intelligence.

Artificial intelligence has entered neurorehabilitation not as a futuristic concept, but as a practical, working tool that is already reshaping how recovery happens. Machine learning systems can now analyze brain signals, movement patterns, speech, cognition, and emotional states with a level of precision that human observation alone cannot achieve. These systems do not replace therapists or neurologists; rather, they enhance their reach, consistency, and personalization. AI makes it possible to identify micro-improvements that would otherwise go unnoticed, to adjust therapy in real time, and to create recovery programs tailored to the unique neural signature of each individual brain. In doing so, AI transforms rehabilitation from a generalized protocol into a living, adaptive process.

Stroke recovery offers one of the clearest examples of this transformation. A stroke disrupts blood flow to specific brain regions, often impairing movement, speech, memory, or emotional regulation. Traditional rehabilitation relies on repetition, intensity, and time—critical elements, but ones limited by human fatigue, scheduling constraints, and subjective assessment. AI systems, by contrast, can track thousands of variables simultaneously, learning how a patient's brain responds to specific exercises, stimuli, and environments. Over time, these systems identify which patterns accelerate recovery and which slow it down, refining therapy with mathematical precision. The result is not simply faster recovery, but deeper and more durable neural reorganization.

What makes AI uniquely powerful in brain healing is its ability to work at scale while remaining deeply individualized. No two brain injuries are identical. Even strokes that affect the same anatomical region can produce vastly different symptoms depending on the individual's prior neural wiring, lifestyle, age, and health history. AI thrives in this complexity. By analyzing large datasets across populations while adapting to individual feedback loops, AI systems bridge the gap between population-level research and personal recovery journeys. They learn not only from one patient, but from millions—compressing decades of clinical insight into actionable, real-time guidance.

Equally important is AI's role in restoring functions once thought irretrievable. Speech recovery, for example, has been revolutionized by AI-powered language models that analyze vocal patterns, cadence, and articulation at granular levels. These systems can detect subtle improvements long before they are audible to human ears, reinforcing progress and guiding targeted exercises. Similarly, AI-driven motor rehabilitation platforms use computer vision and sensor data to retrain movement pathways, helping patients regain coordination, strength, and balance through intelligent feedback rather than brute repetition. In each case, AI acts as a mirror to the brain—reflecting its progress back to itself in a way that strengthens learning and repair.

Beyond physical recovery, AI plays an increasingly critical role in cognitive and emotional healing after brain injury. Stroke survivors frequently experience depression, anxiety, cognitive fog, and emotional dysregulation—symptoms that can be as debilitating as physical impairments. AI-based cognitive training tools, emotional regulation platforms, and adaptive mental health systems now address these dimensions in parallel with physical therapy. By monitoring attention, mood, sleep, and stress patterns, AI helps rebuild not just isolated brain functions, but the integrated systems that support identity, motivation, and quality of life. Healing becomes holistic rather than fragmented.

This book explores how these technologies work, why they are effective, and how they are changing the standard of care for brain injury and stroke recovery. It does not assume technical expertise, nor does it oversimplify the science. Instead, it translates complex neural mechanisms into clear, understandable concepts, showing how algorithms interact with neurons, networks, and behavior to support recovery. You will learn how AI identifies dormant neural pathways, strengthens compensatory circuits, and accelerates relearning through targeted stimulation and feedback. More importantly, you will understand why the brain responds so powerfully to these interventions—and how timing, consistency, and personalization determine outcomes.

The implications extend far beyond stroke recovery alone. Traumatic brain injuries, surgical damage, neurodegenerative conditions, and even age-related cognitive decline all involve disruptions to neural networks that can, in many cases, be retrained. AI offers a framework for ongoing brain maintenance rather than one-time rehabilitation—a shift from reactive medicine to proactive neural health. As these systems continue to evolve, recovery windows once measured in months may extend into years, allowing the brain to continue healing long after conventional therapy ends.

At the same time, this book addresses the ethical and human dimensions of AI-assisted brain healing. Trust, autonomy, data privacy, and emotional connection remain central to recovery. Technology must support human dignity, not override it. AI works best when it empowers patients, therapists, and caregivers with insight rather than replacing human judgment. Throughout this book, you will see how successful neurorehabilitation integrates advanced algorithms with empathy, motivation, and human connection—creating systems that heal both the brain and the person.

AI Brain Healing & Stroke Recovery is ultimately about hope grounded in science. It is about understanding that the brain is not fragile in the way we once believed, but resilient, adaptive, and capable of profound renewal. With AI as a partner, recovery is no longer limited by what clinicians can observe or what patients can repeat. It becomes a collaborative process between human biology and intelligent systems—one that continually learns, adjusts, and improves. As you move through this book, you will discover not only how AI helps the brain repair itself, but why this moment represents one of the most important shifts in neurological care in human history.

*Chapter 1*

# The Science of Brain Repair: How AI Accelerates Neurorehabilitation

Brain healing is not a single event but a continuous biological process driven by adaptation, repetition, and feedback. When a stroke or brain injury occurs, neurons in the affected area may die or lose their ability to communicate effectively. For decades, this loss was believed to be irreversible, leading to rehabilitation models that focused on coping strategies rather than recovery. Modern neuroscience has overturned this assumption by demonstrating that the brain can reorganize itself, rerouting functions through alternative neural pathways when properly stimulated. Artificial intelligence now serves as a catalyst in this process by amplifying the signals that guide neuroplastic change, accelerating learning, and reinforcing recovery at a pace previously unattainable through conventional methods alone.

At the core of AI-assisted brain healing is data. Every movement, word spoken, facial expression, reaction time, and physiological response contains information about how the brain is functioning. Traditional rehabilitation captures only a fraction of this information, relying on periodic evaluations and subjective observation. AI systems, by contrast, continuously collect and analyze high-resolution data streams from sensors, wearables, imaging tools, and digital interfaces. These systems detect subtle trends in neural performance that may be invisible to clinicians, such as micro-improvements in coordination or early signs of cognitive fatigue. By recognizing these patterns, AI adjusts therapy dynamically, ensuring that the brain is challenged without being overwhelmed.

Machine learning models are particularly effective in neurorehabilitation because they thrive in complex, nonlinear environments—exactly the conditions present in the recovering brain. Neural recovery does not follow a straight line. Progress often occurs in bursts, plateaus, or regressions depending on sleep, stress, motivation, and biological timing. AI systems learn from these fluctuations, identifying which interventions produce lasting gains and which merely create temporary improvements. Over time, the algorithm builds a personalized recovery map that reflects how an individual brain learns best, allowing therapy to evolve in sync with the patient rather than following a rigid schedule.

One of the most significant advantages of AI-driven rehabilitation is its ability to target dormant neural circuits. After a stroke, many neurons remain alive but inactive, disconnected from functional networks due to disrupted signaling. AI-powered stimulation systems—combined with guided physical or cognitive tasks—help reactivate these pathways by synchronizing effort with feedback. For example, when a patient attempts to move a weakened limb, AI systems can amplify sensory feedback through visual cues, sound, or haptic signals, reinforcing the brain's association between intention and outcome. This loop strengthens synaptic connections and accelerates relearning.

Timing is another critical factor in brain healing, and AI excels at optimizing it. Neuroplasticity is most responsive during specific windows when the brain is primed for change. These windows vary between individuals and can shift daily based on rest, nutrition, emotional state, and medication. AI systems continuously assess readiness markers—such as reaction speed, error rates, and physiological signals—to determine when therapy will be most effective. Instead of forcing progress on a fixed timetable, AI aligns rehabilitation with the brain's natural rhythms, maximizing efficiency while reducing frustration and burnout.

Speech and language recovery demonstrate how precision matters in neural repair. Language functions involve distributed networks across multiple brain regions, making recovery especially challenging after stroke. AI-driven speech therapy tools analyze phonetics, pacing, syntax, and comprehension in real time, identifying exactly where breakdowns occur. Rather than repeating generic exercises, patients receive targeted prompts that strengthen specific neural connections. The system adapts instantly as performance improves, keeping the brain engaged in the optimal zone of difficulty where learning is strongest.

Cognitive rehabilitation benefits similarly from AI's adaptive capabilities. Attention, memory, and executive function are deeply interconnected, and deficits in one area often affect others. AI-based cognitive training platforms model these relationships, adjusting task complexity to rebuild integrated brain function rather than isolated skills. By monitoring how attention fluctuates during problem-solving or how memory performance changes under stress, AI identifies bottlenecks in cognitive processing and designs exercises that gradually restore balance across neural systems.

Emotional regulation is an equally important but often overlooked component of brain recovery. Stroke survivors frequently experience emotional volatility due to disrupted neural circuits and altered neurotransmitter balance. AI systems that track mood, speech tone, facial expression, and physiological markers can detect emotional dysregulation early, prompting interventions before setbacks escalate. By stabilizing emotional states, AI indirectly supports cognitive and physical recovery, as stress and anxiety are known to inhibit neuroplasticity.

Importantly, AI does not replace human care; it augments it. Therapists, physicians, and caregivers remain essential in providing context, motivation, and empathy. AI acts as an intelligent assistant, offering insights that guide human decision-making rather than dictating it. This partnership allows clinicians to focus on strategy and connection while AI handles continuous measurement and optimization. The result is a rehabilitation model that is both technologically advanced and deeply human.

As AI systems continue to evolve, they are shifting neurorehabilitation from episodic treatment to ongoing brain maintenance. Recovery no longer ends when formal therapy concludes. AI-powered platforms allow patients to continue strengthening neural pathways at home, adapting exercises as the brain improves. This continuity transforms recovery from a limited intervention into a lifelong process of cognitive resilience and neural health. Understanding this foundation is essential for appreciating how AI is redefining what brain healing truly means.

### *Relearning the Signal*

When Daniel woke up in the hospital, the ceiling tiles were the first thing he noticed. They were perfectly aligned, sterile, and unfamiliar. His right arm felt heavy, as if it belonged to someone else. When he tried to speak, the words didn't arrive the way he expected. They hovered just out of reach, fragments of thoughts without sound. A nurse noticed his confusion and spoke gently, but her words came through as echoes rather than meaning. Somewhere in his mind, Daniel understood that something had changed, even if he couldn't yet name it.

The stroke had happened without warning. One moment he was standing in his kitchen making coffee, the next he was on the floor, his body refusing commands it had followed for decades. In the days that followed, doctors explained the damage in careful terms, pointing to images on a screen that showed areas of disrupted blood flow. They spoke about rehabilitation, patience, and gradual improvement. Daniel listened, but what he felt most strongly was uncertainty. He did not know whether his mind would ever feel like his own again.

Rehabilitation began with simple tasks that felt impossibly difficult. Lifting a cup, identifying pictures, repeating basic phrases. Each attempt required intense concentration, and progress was slow. Frustration settled in quietly, heavier than the physical weakness. Daniel worried that effort alone would not be enough, that something fundamental had been lost. Then one afternoon, a therapist introduced a new system—an

AI-guided rehabilitation platform designed to track his movements, speech, and cognitive responses in real time.

At first, Daniel was skeptical. The screen displayed simple exercises, but behind them was a system constantly measuring his reactions. When he reached for an object, sensors tracked not just whether he succeeded, but how his muscles engaged, how quickly he initiated movement, and how consistent his effort was. The feedback was immediate. Visual cues adjusted to guide his motion, encouraging smoother coordination. The system seemed to anticipate his struggles, offering subtle assistance exactly when he needed it.

What surprised Daniel most was how the exercises changed over time. Tasks that once felt overwhelming gradually became manageable, while new challenges appeared just as confidence grew. The system never pushed too far, never allowed boredom to set in. It felt as though someone—or something—was listening to his brain, responding to its signals with patience and precision. For the first time since the stroke, Daniel felt a sense of momentum.

Speech therapy followed a similar pattern. The AI analyzed his pronunciation, rhythm, and word retrieval, highlighting patterns neither Daniel nor his therapist had noticed. When he struggled to form certain sounds, the system adjusted prompts, focusing on specific neural pathways associated with articulation. Progress was measured not in days but in moments—tiny improvements that accumulated into meaningful change. Daniel began to hear his own voice again, hesitant at first, then steadier.

Emotionally, the journey was uneven. Some days brought hope, others exhaustion. The AI system tracked these fluctuations too, noticing changes in his tone and reaction time. On difficult days, exercises shifted toward lighter cognitive tasks, preserving engagement without adding strain. This responsiveness made Daniel feel understood in a way he hadn't expected from technology. It wasn't replacing human support, but it was reinforcing it, offering structure when motivation faltered.

Weeks passed, then months. Daniel regained strength in his arm, clarity in his speech, and confidence in his thinking. Recovery did not mean returning to who he was before, but becoming someone new—someone who understood his brain not as a fixed machine, but as a living system capable of growth. The AI platform continued to evolve alongside him, adapting as his abilities expanded, extending rehabilitation beyond the clinic and into daily life.

One evening, Daniel sat at his kitchen table, holding a cup of coffee with steady hands. The ceiling above him was familiar again, part of a home reclaimed rather than a place remembered. He thought about the invisible work happening inside his brain, the networks reconnecting, the signals strengthening. Healing, he realized, was not a miracle or a single breakthrough. It was a conversation—between effort and feedback, between biology and intelligence, between who he had been and who he was becoming.

*Chapter 2*

# Personalized Neurorehabilitation: How AI Designs a Unique Recovery Path for Every Brain

No two brains are identical, and no two brain injuries unfold in the same way. Even when medical imaging shows damage in similar regions, recovery trajectories can differ dramatically based on prior learning, emotional history, age, physical health, and environmental factors. Traditional neurorehabilitation has long struggled with this variability, relying on standardized protocols designed for the "average" patient. Artificial intelligence changes this paradigm by treating recovery as a personalized system rather than a generalized process, allowing therapy to be shaped continuously around the individual brain rather than forcing the brain to conform to predetermined expectations.

Personalized neurorehabilitation begins with comprehensive data capture. AI systems gather information from multiple layers of brain function simultaneously, including movement patterns, speech dynamics, cognitive performance, emotional responses, and physiological signals such as heart rate variability and sleep cycles. This multidimensional view allows

AI to construct a functional profile of how a brain is operating in real time. Rather than focusing solely on deficits, the system identifies preserved strengths, compensatory pathways, and latent capacities that can be leveraged during recovery. In doing so, AI reframes rehabilitation from repairing what is broken to amplifying what still works.

Machine learning models excel at identifying hidden relationships within complex datasets. In neurorehabilitation, this means uncovering how subtle variables interact to influence recovery outcomes. For example, AI may detect that a patient's speech improves after physical therapy sessions or that cognitive performance declines when sleep quality drops below a certain threshold. These insights allow rehabilitation plans to be adjusted holistically rather than in isolation. Therapy becomes an integrated ecosystem in which physical, cognitive, and emotional interventions reinforce one another instead of competing for limited neural resources.

One of the most transformative aspects of AI personalization is adaptive difficulty calibration. Effective brain retraining requires tasks to remain within a narrow window of challenge—difficult enough to stimulate learning, but not so difficult that they induce stress or disengagement. Human therapists approximate this balance through experience and observation, but AI refines it through continuous measurement. As performance fluctuates, the system adjusts task complexity instantly, ensuring the brain remains in an optimal learning state. This responsiveness significantly accelerates synaptic strengthening and skill reacquisition.

AI-driven personalization also addresses a longstanding limitation in rehabilitation: inconsistency. Human-delivered therapy varies based on time constraints, fatigue, and subjective interpretation. AI systems, by contrast, apply consistent evaluation criteria while adapting content dynamically. Every repetition is measured, every response logged, and every adjustment informed by prior outcomes. This consistency does not remove the human element; instead, it provides therapists with objective insights that support more informed clinical decisions. The result is a partnership in which human expertise guides strategy while AI manages precision.

Another critical dimension of personalization lies in motivation and engagement. Recovery requires sustained effort over long periods, often accompanied by frustration and emotional fatigue. AI systems monitor engagement signals such as reaction time variability, error patterns, and behavioral hesitation to assess motivation levels. When disengagement is detected, exercises can shift format, pacing, or sensory modality to re-engage the brain. This adaptability transforms therapy from a rigid routine into an evolving experience that maintains psychological resilience alongside neurological progress.

Language recovery highlights the importance of individualized neural mapping. Speech is distributed across networks that vary significantly between individuals. AI systems analyze speech output at granular levels, identifying which linguistic components—such as phonological processing, semantic retrieval, or syntactic construction—are most affected. Therapy then targets these specific components rather than applying generalized speech drills. As recovery progresses, AI continuously remaps neural changes, ensuring that therapy evolves alongside the brain's reorganization rather than lagging behind it.

Personalized neurorehabilitation extends beyond clinical settings into daily life. AI-powered platforms enable continuous reinforcement of recovery activities at home, integrating rehabilitation into routine tasks. This continuity is essential for long-term outcomes, as neuroplastic change depends on frequent, meaningful activation rather than isolated therapy sessions. By embedding recovery into everyday contexts, AI transforms rehabilitation from an episodic intervention into a sustained lifestyle adaptation that supports ongoing brain health. Ethically, personalization raises important considerations around autonomy and trust. Effective AI-driven rehabilitation respects patient agency by making progress transparent and goals collaborative. Rather than imposing opaque algorithms, successful systems communicate insights in understandable ways, empowering patients to participate actively in their recovery. Personalization becomes not just a technical feature, but a relational one—strengthening the connection between patient, clinician, and technology.

Ultimately, personalized neurorehabilitation represents a shift from reactive care to responsive care. Instead of responding only to observable deficits, AI anticipates needs, adapts strategies, and supports the brain's intrinsic capacity for repair. This approach acknowledges that healing is not linear, uniform, or predictable—but it is learnable. By designing recovery paths as unique as the brains they serve, AI redefines what meaningful rehabilitation looks like in the modern era.

### *The Shape of Progress*

Maria had always believed discipline could solve almost anything. Before her stroke, she managed projects, schedules, and people with calm efficiency. When rehabilitation began, she approached it the same way, determined to follow every instruction perfectly. Yet weeks passed with uneven progress. Some days she spoke clearly, other days words tangled unexpectedly. Her left hand regained strength, then seemed to forget what it had learned. The inconsistency unsettled her more than the difficulty itself.

Her therapist introduced an AI-based rehabilitation system designed to personalize recovery. At first, Maria saw it as another tool, nothing more. But the system quickly revealed patterns she had not noticed. It showed that her speech improved after emotionally positive interactions and declined when she felt rushed. It revealed that fine motor control strengthened in the afternoon but weakened in the morning. These insights reframed her frustration. The problem was not effort; it was timing and alignment.

As therapy continued, exercises shifted subtly. On days when Maria's attention wavered, tasks became shorter but more frequent. When emotional fatigue surfaced, cognitive challenges eased while physical movement increased. The system adapted without judgment, responding to her brain rather than her expectations. For the first time, Maria felt that recovery was meeting her where she was, not where she was supposed to be.

The personalization extended into her home. The system suggested simple daily activities that reinforced therapy—folding laundry in specific ways, reading aloud at particular times, practicing movement during moments of calm. These tasks felt natural, integrated rather than imposed. Progress no longer belonged only to the clinic; it lived in her daily routine. Gradually, Maria stopped measuring success by comparison to her past self. Instead, she noticed patterns of growth—how clarity followed rest, how confidence improved with consistency. The AI system continued to learn alongside her, adjusting as her brain changed. Recovery became less about returning to who she had been and more about shaping who she was becoming.

One afternoon, Maria caught herself explaining a concept clearly and without hesitation. The moment passed quietly, unnoticed by anyone else. But she recognized it as progress shaped by understanding rather than force. Healing, she realized, had a shape—one defined not by speed or perfection, but by responsiveness and care.

*Chapter 3*

# Human–AI Collaboration in Brain Recovery: The Therapist, the Patient, and the Algorithm

Brain healing does not occur in isolation, nor can it be reduced to technology alone. While artificial intelligence provides unprecedented analytical power, recovery ultimately emerges from a collaboration between human intention, biological adaptability, and intelligent systems. The most successful neurorehabilitation models recognize that AI is not a replacement for clinicians or caregivers, but a partner that enhances their ability to guide, motivate, and personalize healing. Understanding this collaborative dynamic is essential for appreciating how AI transforms recovery without diminishing the human element at its core.

At the center of this collaboration is the patient's active participation. Neuroplastic change depends on effort, attention, and repetition—factors that cannot be automated. AI supports these processes by creating structured feedback loops that translate effort into measurable progress. When a patient attempts a movement or cognitive task, the algorithm captures nuanced data about the attempt, reinforcing successful patterns and gently correcting ineffective ones. This immediate feedback strengthens the brain's learning signals, making effort more meaningful and reducing the uncertainty that often undermines motivation during recovery.

Clinicians play a critical role in interpreting and contextualizing AI insights. While algorithms excel at detecting patterns, they do not understand personal narratives, emotional history, or social context without human guidance. Therapists integrate AI-generated data with clinical judgment, adjusting goals and interventions based on factors such as patient mood, life circumstances, and long-term priorities. This integration transforms therapy sessions from reactive problem-solving into proactive strategy-building, where decisions are informed by both quantitative evidence and human understanding.

AI also reshapes the role of therapists by reducing cognitive load. Continuous monitoring and data analysis free clinicians from manual tracking, allowing them to focus on high-value activities such as coaching, emotional support, and creative problem-solving. Rather than spending time documenting progress after the fact, therapists can engage more deeply with patients in the moment, using AI insights to guide conversations and reinforce successes. This shift enhances therapeutic relationships, strengthening trust and collaboration. Caregivers and family members become part of the recovery ecosystem through AI-enabled transparency. Many AI platforms provide simplified progress summaries that make neural recovery visible and understandable. These insights help caregivers support rehabilitation efforts more effectively, aligning daily routines with therapeutic goals. When caregivers understand how sleep, stress, and engagement influence recovery, they can create environments that reinforce healing rather than inadvertently hinder it. AI thus extends rehabilitation beyond clinical boundaries into the social fabric of the patient's life.

Ethical design is central to effective human–AI collaboration. Transparency, consent, and data security are not optional features but foundational principles. Patients must understand how AI systems work, what data is collected, and how insights are used. Empowerment arises when individuals feel informed and in control of their recovery journey rather than monitored or judged by opaque systems. Ethical AI fosters trust, which is itself a powerful facilitator of neuroplastic change.

Another essential aspect of collaboration is adaptability across recovery stages. Early rehabilitation often emphasizes basic functions, while later stages focus on refinement and resilience. AI systems evolve alongside these stages, shifting from intensive guidance to subtle optimization. This adaptability prevents stagnation and supports long-term brain health beyond initial recovery. Human oversight ensures that technological adjustments align with evolving personal goals, preserving autonomy and relevance.

Human–AI collaboration also mitigates the emotional challenges of recovery. Frustration, grief, and identity shifts are common after brain injury. AI systems can detect emotional stress markers, but empathetic response requires human connection. Therapists use AI insights to time encouragement, adjust expectations, and validate experiences. This synergy transforms data into compassion, ensuring that recovery addresses emotional as well as neurological needs.

Ultimately, collaboration defines the future of neurorehabilitation. AI provides clarity, consistency, and adaptability; humans provide meaning, motivation, and care. Together, they create recovery systems that honor both the complexity of the brain and the individuality of the person. Understanding this partnership reframes AI not as an external force acting on the brain, but as an extension of human intention—guiding healing through insight, responsiveness, and shared purpose.

*Holding the Line*

When Thomas began rehabilitation, he felt caught between hope and exhaustion. His therapist, Elena, had guided patients through recovery for years, but this case felt different. An AI-assisted platform tracked Thomas's progress continuously, providing streams of data that revealed patterns she had never been able to see so clearly before. At first, the volume of information felt overwhelming. Then Elena realized the data was not replacing her intuition—it was sharpening it.

During sessions, Thomas worked through exercises while the AI system quietly analyzed his movements and speech. Elena watched his posture, his expressions, the moments when his focus drifted. The system highlighted subtle improvements, confirming her observations and occasionally challenging her assumptions. When progress slowed, Elena used the insights to adjust therapy rather than push harder. The collaboration felt natural, as if the technology were another set of attentive eyes rather than a detached machine.

Thomas noticed the difference too. Feedback was immediate and specific. When frustration surfaced, Elena explained what the system showed—not as a judgment, but as information. Understanding transformed his mindset. Setbacks became data points rather than failures. Effort regained meaning because it was visible, measurable, and shared.

At home, Thomas's family accessed simplified updates that explained how daily habits influenced recovery. They adjusted routines, supported rest, and celebrated small milestones together. Recovery became a collective effort, guided by insight rather than guesswork. The AI system connected their actions to Thomas's progress, strengthening motivation across the household.

Over time, Thomas's abilities improved steadily. The AI adapted, offering less guidance as confidence grew. Elena shifted her role from instructor to coach, focusing on resilience and long-term goals. Collaboration evolved rather than ended. Recovery was no longer about regaining what was lost, but about building strength through partnership.

One afternoon, Thomas completed a task smoothly and paused, surprised by how natural it felt. Elena smiled, not because the system had predicted the outcome, but because they had arrived there together. Technology had not led the way—it had held the line, steady and responsive, while human effort and care did the rest.

*Chapter 4*

# Timing, Intensity, and Feedback: How AI Optimizes the Brain's Windows for Healing

Brain recovery is governed not only by what rehabilitation activities are performed, but by when and how they are delivered. Neuroplasticity does not operate at a constant rate; instead, it fluctuates based on biological readiness, emotional state, fatigue, and environmental conditions. Traditional rehabilitation models often overlook this variability, applying therapy according to fixed schedules rather than neural responsiveness. Artificial intelligence fundamentally alters this limitation by identifying and exploiting the brain's optimal windows for change, ensuring that effort is applied when it will produce the greatest neurological return.

At the biological level, neuroplasticity is influenced by neurotransmitter availability, synaptic sensitivity, and neural network excitability. These factors vary throughout the day and across stages of recovery. AI systems continuously monitor behavioral and physiological indicators—such as reaction time, accuracy, heart rate variability, and engagement patterns—to infer when the brain is most receptive to learning.

By aligning therapy with these windows, AI increases the efficiency of rehabilitation, allowing fewer repetitions to generate stronger neural connections.

Intensity is another critical variable that AI refines with precision. Too little challenge fails to stimulate neural growth, while excessive intensity triggers stress responses that inhibit learning. Human therapists estimate appropriate intensity based on observation and experience, but AI quantifies it. Algorithms track micro-level changes in performance to determine when a task is optimally difficult. As soon as a task becomes too easy or too taxing, the system adjusts parameters such as speed, complexity, or sensory input. This constant recalibration keeps the brain operating in its most productive learning zone.

Feedback plays a central role in reinforcing neural adaptation. The brain learns through consequences—signals that confirm or correct its actions. AI enhances this process by delivering immediate, multimodal feedback that strengthens neural associations. Visual cues, auditory signals, and tactile responses are synchronized with performance, creating rich feedback loops that accelerate synaptic reinforcement. This immediacy reduces ambiguity, helping the brain distinguish successful patterns from ineffective ones more clearly than delayed verbal feedback alone. AI also addresses a subtle but powerful barrier to recovery: delayed awareness of progress. Many patients experience discouragement because improvements occur gradually and are difficult to perceive. AI systems capture incremental gains that might otherwise go unnoticed, translating them into tangible metrics or visualizations. Seeing progress reinforces motivation, which itself enhances neuroplasticity by increasing attention and emotional engagement. In this way, feedback does not merely reflect recovery—it actively drives it.

Another advantage of AI-optimized timing is fatigue management. Neural fatigue undermines learning by reducing signal clarity and increasing error rates. AI detects early signs of fatigue through changes in performance variability and physiological markers, adjusting therapy accordingly. Instead of pushing through diminishing returns, the system shifts to complementary activities or recommends rest. This approach respects the brain's limits, preserving energy for future learning and preventing setbacks associated with overtraining.

The integration of timing, intensity, and feedback transforms rehabilitation into a dynamic dialogue with the brain. Rather than imposing a static program, AI listens to neural responses and replies with precisely calibrated challenges. This responsiveness accelerates recovery while reducing frustration and burnout. Therapy becomes adaptive rather than prescriptive, evolving as the brain heals and reorganizes.

Importantly, these optimizations extend beyond structured therapy sessions. AI-enabled tools can guide daily activities, suggesting when to practice skills, when to rest, and when to engage in cognitively demanding tasks. This guidance embeds recovery into the rhythms of everyday life, reinforcing neural changes continuously rather than episodically. Over time, this integration supports sustained improvement and long-term brain resilience.

The ethical dimension of optimization requires transparency and collaboration. Patients must understand how timing and intensity decisions are made, ensuring trust and autonomy. When AI recommendations are communicated clearly and adjusted in partnership with clinicians and patients, optimization becomes empowering rather than controlling. The brain heals best when effort is informed, intentional, and aligned with its natural rhythms.

Ultimately, optimizing timing, intensity, and feedback represents one of AI's greatest contributions to brain healing. By respecting the brain's dynamic nature, AI transforms rehabilitation from a repetitive process into a responsive system. Healing becomes more efficient, more humane, and more sustainable—guided not by rigid schedules, but by the brain's own signals for growth.

*The Right Moment*

Evelyn had always believed that more effort meant better results. After her stroke, she applied this belief relentlessly, pushing herself through every exercise with determination bordering on stubbornness. Yet progress felt uneven. Some sessions left her energized, others drained and discouraged. She could not understand why the same effort produced different outcomes. The inconsistency gnawed at her confidence.

When her rehabilitation team introduced an AI-guided system, Evelyn was skeptical. She expected another set of exercises, another schedule to follow. Instead, the system began by observing. It tracked her reaction times, her accuracy, even subtle pauses that reflected hesitation or fatigue. Over several sessions, patterns emerged. The AI revealed that her best progress occurred during mid-morning sessions, while late afternoons often led to frustration and mistakes.

Therapy shifted accordingly. Exercises became more demanding during optimal windows and gentler when her brain showed signs of fatigue. Feedback arrived instantly—visual cues brightened when movements aligned correctly, sounds softened when tension increased. The system adjusted without commentary, allowing Evelyn to focus on the task rather than the rules. Gradually, effort felt purposeful again.

At home, Evelyn noticed changes too. The system suggested practicing certain skills shortly after rest and avoiding others when tired. She learned to recognize her own rhythms, understanding that recovery was not about constant exertion but about timing. Progress accelerated, not because she worked harder, but because she worked smarter.

One afternoon, Evelyn completed a complex task smoothly and without strain. The ease surprised her. She realized that healing was less about force and more about alignment—meeting the brain when it was ready. The AI had not replaced her determination; it had refined it. Recovery, she learned, was about choosing the right moment and honoring it.

*Chapter 5*

# Beyond the Clinic: AI, Home-Based Recovery, and Long-Term Brain Resilience

One of the most significant limitations of traditional neurorehabilitation is that it is often confined to clinical environments and finite timelines. Therapy sessions occur a few times per week, progress is evaluated intermittently, and formal rehabilitation eventually ends—even though the brain's capacity for adaptation continues long after discharge. Artificial intelligence breaks this constraint by extending recovery beyond the clinic and into daily life, transforming rehabilitation from a short-term intervention into a sustained process of brain resilience and long-term healing.

The brain does not distinguish between "therapy time" and "real life." Neural networks strengthen through repeated, meaningful activation regardless of setting. AI-powered home-based recovery systems leverage this principle by embedding therapeutic guidance into everyday activities. Through mobile applications, wearable sensors, and adaptive digital platforms, AI monitors performance and engagement during routine tasks such as walking, speaking, reading, or problem-solving. These systems identify opportunities for reinforcement, subtly guiding behavior in ways that promote continued neural reorganization without disrupting normal life.

Continuity is critical for durable neuroplastic change. While clinical therapy establishes foundational skills, long-term recovery depends on consistent practice over months or years. AI systems provide this continuity by maintaining personalized rehabilitation plans that evolve alongside the recovering brain. As abilities improve, exercises adapt automatically, preventing stagnation and ensuring that neural challenges remain relevant. This sustained engagement reduces the risk of regression and supports gradual refinement of function rather than abrupt plateaus.

Home-based AI rehabilitation also democratizes access to care. Geographic barriers, financial constraints, and limited clinical availability often restrict therapy duration. AI platforms reduce reliance on in-person sessions by providing high-quality guidance remotely, enabling patients to continue recovery regardless of location. Clinicians remain involved through periodic reviews and oversight, but the day-to-day reinforcement occurs independently. This model expands rehabilitation capacity while preserving clinical expertise where it matters most. Long-term brain resilience involves more than restoring lost function; it requires protecting neural health against future decline. AI systems monitor lifestyle factors that influence brain recovery, including sleep quality, stress levels, physical activity, and cognitive load. By correlating these factors with performance trends, AI offers actionable insights that help individuals make choices supporting neural stability. Recovery thus becomes proactive rather than reactive, focused on maintaining gains rather than merely reclaiming what was lost.

Another advantage of AI-supported home recovery is identity reconstruction. After brain injury or stroke, individuals often struggle with a disrupted sense of self. Returning to meaningful activities—work, hobbies, relationships—plays a vital role in psychological healing. AI systems support this transition by integrating recovery tasks into personally relevant contexts. Rather than practicing abstract exercises, individuals relearn skills through activities that align with their values and goals, reinforcing both neural and emotional restoration.

Caregiver involvement becomes more effective through AI-enabled transparency. Simplified dashboards and progress summaries help families understand recovery trajectories, reinforcing supportive behaviors at home. When caregivers see how daily routines influence outcomes, they become active participants in sustaining progress. This shared understanding reduces frustration and aligns expectations, creating environments conducive to long-term healing.

Ethical considerations are especially important as recovery moves into private spaces. AI systems must prioritize privacy, consent, and user control. Successful home-based rehabilitation platforms are designed to be supportive rather than intrusive, offering guidance without surveillance. When individuals retain autonomy over how and when technology engages, trust is preserved, and long-term adoption becomes sustainable.

Ultimately, AI extends brain healing from an event into a lifestyle. Recovery does not end when therapy concludes; it continues as the brain adapts to new challenges and environments. By supporting home-based recovery and long-term resilience, AI redefines success in neurorehabilitation—not as a return to baseline, but as the cultivation of a brain capable of ongoing growth, adaptation, and stability over time.

### *The Quiet Continuation*

After being discharged from formal therapy, Jonathan expected recovery to slow. Without scheduled sessions and constant supervision, he feared progress would fade. His therapist introduced him to an AI-supported home recovery platform designed to continue adapting alongside him. At first, Jonathan treated it cautiously, unsure how technology could replace structured care.

The system blended quietly into his routine. It suggested short exercises integrated into daily activities—walking with intentional pacing, speaking aloud while cooking, focusing attention during reading. Sensors tracked subtle performance changes, adjusting guidance without interruption. Jonathan noticed that recovery no longer felt like an obligation; it became part of how he lived.

Weeks passed, and improvement continued. The system highlighted patterns Jonathan hadn't noticed, showing how rest improved clarity and how stress affected coordination. These insights helped him make small adjustments that produced steady gains. Recovery felt less fragile, more grounded.

Family members followed his progress through simple summaries that explained trends rather than numbers. Support became collaborative rather than anxious. Jonathan regained confidence not because therapy was watching, but because understanding replaced uncertainty.

One evening, Jonathan realized he had completed an entire

day without consciously thinking about recovery. Skills flowed naturally, integrated into his identity. Healing had not stopped—it had simply moved into the background. The AI system remained present but unobtrusive, supporting growth without defining it. Jonathan understood then that recovery was not something to finish, but something to live. With guidance woven into daily life, the brain continued to strengthen quietly, resilient and ready for what came next.

*Chapter 6*

# Cognition, Emotion, and Identity: How AI Supports Whole-Brain Recovery After Injury

Brain healing is often discussed in terms of physical recovery—movement restored, speech regained, coordination improved—but true neurological recovery extends far beyond these visible milestones. Stroke and brain injury frequently disrupt cognition, emotional regulation, and personal identity, altering how individuals think, feel, and relate to the world. These changes can be subtle or profound, temporary or persistent, but they shape the lived experience of recovery as much as any physical impairment. Artificial intelligence plays a critical role in addressing these deeper dimensions by supporting whole-brain recovery rather than isolated functional repair.

Cognitive disruption after brain injury often manifests as difficulty with attention, memory, planning, or decision-making. These functions rely on distributed neural networks that must work in coordination to support daily life. Traditional cognitive rehabilitation typically targets these skills through standardized exercises, but such approaches may overlook individual patterns of disruption. AI systems analyze cognitive performance across multiple domains simultaneously, identifying how deficits interact rather than treating them in isolation. This systems-level perspective allows rehabilitation to rebuild cognitive coherence rather than fragmented skills.

Emotional regulation is equally central to recovery. Damage to neural pathways involved in mood, impulse control, and stress response can lead to emotional volatility, depression, or anxiety. These changes are not merely psychological reactions to injury; they are neurological consequences that influence motivation, learning capacity, and neuroplastic potential. AI-driven emotional monitoring tools detect subtle indicators of dysregulation—changes in speech tone, reaction time variability, physiological stress markers—and respond by adjusting cognitive load or therapeutic intensity. Stabilizing emotional states creates a neurological environment conducive to learning and repair.

Identity reconstruction is one of the most complex challenges following brain injury. Individuals may feel disconnected from their previous sense of self, struggling with altered abilities, priorities, or emotional responses. AI-supported recovery addresses this challenge by integrating rehabilitation into meaningful contexts rather than abstract tasks. By aligning exercises with personal goals, interests, and values, AI helps individuals rebuild a coherent narrative of who they are becoming rather than who they have lost. Recovery shifts from restoration to reinvention, guided by intention rather than nostalgia.

The interplay between cognition and emotion is particularly important in neuroplastic change. Stress and frustration impair learning by disrupting attention and neurotransmitter balance, while positive engagement enhances synaptic strengthening. AI systems optimize this balance by monitoring engagement signals and adjusting task difficulty to maintain a productive emotional state. When cognitive challenges align with emotional readiness, learning becomes more efficient and sustainable. This alignment transforms rehabilitation from a struggle into a collaborative exploration of capacity.

AI also supports metacognition—the ability to understand and regulate one's own thinking. Many individuals experience confusion or self-doubt during recovery, unsure whether difficulties reflect permanent limitations or temporary disruptions. AI-generated insights provide clarity by distinguishing between variability and trend, helping individuals interpret their experiences accurately. This understanding reduces anxiety and fosters patience, reinforcing long-term commitment to recovery. Social cognition and communication are additional dimensions of whole-brain healing. Brain injury can affect empathy, social timing, and conversational flow, creating challenges in relationships even when speech mechanics improve. AI-assisted social cognition training analyzes interaction patterns and provides feedback that refines timing, tone, and responsiveness. These subtle adjustments restore social confidence, enabling reintegration into personal and professional communities.

Ethical considerations are paramount when addressing cognition, emotion, and identity through AI. Systems must respect individuality, avoid pathologizing normal emotional responses, and prioritize informed consent. Successful AI-supported recovery empowers individuals rather than defining them by metrics. Technology serves as a mirror for growth, not a label for limitation.

Ultimately, whole-brain recovery recognizes that healing is not complete until individuals feel cognitively capable, emotionally stable, and personally whole. AI enables this integration by supporting the invisible dimensions of recovery that shape quality of life. By addressing cognition, emotion, and identity together, AI transforms rehabilitation into a process of re-inhabiting the self—restoring not just function, but meaning.

*Becoming Again*

After the stroke, Nathan's greatest fear was not that he would walk differently or speak more slowly. It was that he no longer recognized himself. Conversations felt harder to follow, emotions surfaced unexpectedly, and decisions that once came easily now required effort. Friends assured him that recovery took time, but Nathan worried that time alone would not restore what felt fundamentally altered.

When his rehabilitation team introduced an AI-supported cognitive and emotional recovery program, Nathan approached it cautiously. The system did not begin with demanding tasks. Instead, it observed—how he responded to questions, how his attention shifted, how his tone changed under pressure. Gradually, it began tailoring exercises that challenged his thinking without overwhelming him. Tasks adjusted fluidly, maintaining focus while avoiding frustration.

Emotionally, Nathan noticed subtle shifts. On days when anxiety crept in, cognitive demands softened, allowing engagement without strain. When confidence returned, challenges increased. The system seemed to understand his rhythms, responding to emotional cues he had not yet learned to recognize himself. For the first time, recovery felt attuned rather than imposed.

Over weeks, Nathan's thinking grew clearer. More importantly, his sense of self stabilized. The AI-guided program integrated tasks related to his interests—problem-solving scenarios tied to work he cared about, conversations reflecting social contexts he valued. Recovery stopped feeling like rehearsal for life and became life itself.

One evening, Nathan found himself laughing easily during a conversation, fully present and engaged. The moment surprised him not because it felt extraordinary, but because it felt ordinary again. He realized that healing had not erased change; it had woven change into a new coherence. Identity was not restored by returning to the past, but by growing forward with understanding.

Nathan understood then that recovery was not about reclaiming a former version of himself. It was about becoming again—supported by insight, patience, and systems designed to honor the whole brain. With that realization, the future felt navigable, not because it was familiar, but because he was ready to meet it.

*Chapter 7*

# From Recovery to Reintegration: How AI Supports the Return to Work, Purpose, and Daily Mastery

The later stages of brain recovery are often the most underestimated and the least supported. While early rehabilitation focuses on restoring basic functions, long-term success depends on reintegration—the ability to return to meaningful roles, responsibilities, and environments with confidence and competence. This phase requires far more than physical or cognitive capacity; it demands adaptability, endurance, emotional regulation, and contextual intelligence. Artificial intelligence plays a critical role in this transition by bridging the gap between clinical recovery and real-world performance, transforming regained ability into functional mastery.

Reintegration challenges the brain in ways that controlled therapy environments cannot fully simulate. Workplaces, social settings, and daily responsibilities introduce unpredictability, multitasking demands, and emotional complexity. Traditional rehabilitation often ends before individuals are exposed to these conditions, leaving a gap between capability and application. AI-supported reintegration addresses this gap by modeling real-world cognitive loads and gradually introducing complexity in a measured, adaptive way. Instead of abrupt exposure, individuals experience progressive challenges aligned with their readiness.

AI systems analyze performance not only in isolation but within context. For example, returning to work requires sustained attention, decision-making under pressure, and efficient task switching. AI monitors these functions during simulated or real activities, identifying stress points and inefficiencies. By isolating specific breakdowns—such as cognitive fatigue after prolonged focus or errors during multitasking—AI enables targeted interventions that refine performance rather than repeating foundational training unnecessarily.

Endurance is a central component of reintegration. Cognitive stamina, unlike physical strength, is difficult to measure subjectively. AI systems quantify endurance through metrics such as sustained accuracy, reaction time consistency, and recovery after exertion. These insights inform pacing strategies that prevent burnout while extending capacity gradually. Reintegration becomes sustainable rather than overwhelming, allowing individuals to rebuild confidence through consistency. Emotional resilience is equally essential. Returning to familiar environments can trigger anxiety, self-doubt, or fear of failure. AI-assisted emotional monitoring detects stress responses early, enabling proactive adjustments in workload or support. By stabilizing emotional states, AI preserves cognitive resources needed for performance. This integration ensures that reintegration supports psychological safety alongside productivity.

Identity plays a powerful role in this phase of recovery. Individuals often measure success by their ability to resume previous roles, but rigid attachment to past identities can hinder adaptation. AI-supported reintegration reframes success by focusing on functional effectiveness rather than exact replication of prior performance. By highlighting progress and adaptability, AI helps individuals redefine competence in ways that honor growth rather than loss.

Social reintegration also benefits from AI-guided feedback. Communication timing, tone, and responsiveness are critical in professional and personal settings. AI systems analyze interaction patterns, offering subtle guidance that refines social performance without scripting behavior. These refinements restore confidence in social engagement, reducing isolation and supporting collaborative reintegration.

Long-term monitoring distinguishes reintegration from short-term return. AI systems continue to observe performance trends over time, identifying early signs of overload or regression. This ongoing support allows for timely adjustments, preventing setbacks that might otherwise derail progress. Reintegration becomes a dynamic process rather than a one-time milestone.

Ethical reintegration requires respect for autonomy and dignity. AI systems must support choice rather than impose standards. Successful reintegration tools empower individuals to set goals, adjust pacing, and define success on their own terms. Technology becomes an ally in reclaiming agency rather than a measure of worth.

Ultimately, reintegration represents the culmination of brain healing—not because recovery ends, but because it becomes fully integrated into life. AI ensures that regained abilities translate into meaningful participation, enabling individuals to move forward with competence, resilience, and purpose. Recovery evolves into mastery, supported by systems designed to honor the complexity of real life.

### *Crossing the Threshold*

For months, Daniel had imagined returning to work as the final proof that recovery was complete. Yet when the opportunity arrived, confidence wavered. The office felt louder than he remembered, the pace faster, the expectations heavier. Tasks he once handled effortlessly now required conscious effort. The gap between rehabilitation and reality became painfully clear.

His recovery team introduced an AI-supported reintegration program designed to bridge that gap. Rather than throwing him into full responsibility, the system simulated work-like challenges—extended focus sessions, decision-making under mild pressure, task switching with increasing complexity. Performance data revealed patterns Daniel had not recognized: cognitive fatigue surfaced after sustained meetings, while accuracy dipped during rapid transitions.

With this insight, reintegration became strategic. Workdays were structured around optimal performance windows, with gradual increases in responsibility. The AI system monitored endurance and emotional stress, adjusting challenges before overwhelm set in. Daniel felt supported without being shielded, challenged without being pushed beyond capacity.

Social interactions proved unexpectedly difficult. Conversations required more attention than before, and Daniel worried about appearing slow or uncertain. The AI system analyzed communication patterns, offering feedback that refined pacing and tone. Small adjustments restored confidence, making interactions feel natural again. Weeks passed, and routines stabilized. Daniel no longer measured success by comparison to his past self, but by consistency and effectiveness. Work felt manageable, even satisfying. The threshold he had feared crossing now felt behind him, not because he had returned unchanged, but because he had adapted intelligently.

One evening, Daniel left the office with a quiet sense of accomplishment. Recovery had not ended—it had matured. Supported by insight, patience, and adaptive systems, he had crossed from healing into living. The future no longer felt like a test, but a continuation.

*Chapter 8*

# Adaptive Intelligence and the Future of Neurorehabilitation: How AI Evolves With the Healing Brain

As brain recovery progresses, the nature of rehabilitation must evolve as well. Early stages emphasize restoration and stabilization, while later stages demand refinement, resilience, and adaptability. One of artificial intelligence's most profound contributions to neurorehabilitation is its capacity to evolve alongside the brain it supports. Unlike static therapeutic protocols, AI systems are designed to learn continuously, recalibrating their strategies as neural patterns change. This adaptability positions AI not merely as a rehabilitation tool, but as a long-term partner in neurological health.

The recovering brain is not a fixed target. Neural networks reorganize, compensate, and strengthen in nonlinear ways, often producing unexpected plateaus or breakthroughs. AI systems thrive in these conditions because they are not bound to predetermined assumptions about how recovery "should" unfold. Machine learning models analyze ongoing data streams, updating predictions and interventions as new information emerges. This capacity allows therapy to remain aligned with the brain's current state rather than its historical profile.

Adaptive intelligence also enables AI to detect transitions between recovery phases. Subtle shifts in performance patterns—such as increased variability preceding improvement—can signal readiness for new challenges. AI systems recognize these signals earlier than human observation alone, introducing changes that capitalize on emerging capacity. This proactive adjustment prevents stagnation and sustains momentum, ensuring that progress continues even when visible gains appear minimal.

As rehabilitation advances, the focus often shifts from reacquiring basic skills to optimizing performance under complexity. AI supports this transition by introducing layered challenges that integrate multiple cognitive and motor demands. Rather than training isolated functions, adaptive systems simulate real-world conditions that require coordination, prioritization, and flexibility. This prepares the brain for environments that cannot be fully controlled, reinforcing robustness rather than perfection.

Long-term adaptation also addresses variability inherent in daily life. Stress, fatigue, and environmental changes influence neural performance, even years after injury. AI systems account for this variability by adjusting expectations and recommendations dynamically. Instead of interpreting fluctuations as failure, adaptive models contextualize them within broader trends, preserving confidence and guiding sustainable behavior. This perspective reframes recovery as a living process rather than a linear trajectory.

The future of neurorehabilitation increasingly involves hybrid systems that integrate AI with emerging neurotechnologies. Brain–computer interfaces, noninvasive stimulation tools, and advanced imaging technologies generate data that AI can synthesize into actionable insights. While this book focuses on current applications, understanding AI's adaptive foundation prepares readers to engage thoughtfully with future innovations. The core principle remains the same: technology must respond to the brain, not dictate it.

Ethical foresight becomes increasingly important as AI systems grow more autonomous. Adaptive intelligence must remain transparent, explainable, and accountable. Individuals should understand how systems learn, why adjustments occur, and how to override recommendations when necessary. Adaptive AI enhances recovery only when trust is maintained and human agency preserved. Ethical design ensures that evolution serves empowerment rather than dependence. Adaptation also extends to lifespan brain health. Recovery from stroke or injury often marks the beginning of heightened awareness of cognitive well-being. AI systems that continue monitoring and guiding behavior beyond rehabilitation support long-term neuroprotection. By identifying early signs of cognitive decline or stress-related impairment, adaptive systems enable preventative interventions that preserve brain health over time. Rehabilitation thus becomes a gateway to lifelong neural stewardship.

Ultimately, adaptive intelligence represents a philosophical shift in how recovery is understood. Healing is no longer a finite project with a defined endpoint, but an evolving relationship between brain, behavior, and environment. AI's capacity to learn alongside the brain mirrors the brain's own plasticity, creating a partnership rooted in responsiveness and growth. In this model, recovery does not conclude—it matures, supported by systems designed to evolve as life unfolds.

### *The Long View*

Years after his stroke, Marcus no longer thought of himself as "recovering." He had returned to work, rebuilt routines, and adapted to subtle changes in how his mind processed information. Yet challenges still appeared—days when focus slipped, moments when stress disrupted clarity. What surprised him was not the presence of these fluctuations, but how differently he now responded to them.

Marcus continued using an AI-supported cognitive platform introduced during rehabilitation. Unlike earlier stages, the system no longer emphasized structured exercises. Instead, it observed patterns across his daily life—how sleep affected concentration, how stress influenced decision-making, how sustained effort shaped fatigue. Feedback arrived gently, often as suggestions rather than instructions.

When Marcus faced increased demands at work, the system adjusted expectations, recommending pacing strategies rather than intensified effort. It recognized patterns Marcus himself had not yet articulated. Variability became information rather than threat. Confidence grew not because performance was perfect, but because it was understood.

One month, Marcus noticed that tasks requiring rapid switching felt harder. The AI system correlated this change with prolonged stress and reduced rest, suggesting adjustments before frustration set in. With small changes, clarity returned. The system evolved as he did, reflecting a partnership rather than supervision.

Looking back, Marcus realized that recovery had not ended when therapy stopped. It had transformed into awareness, adaptability, and resilience. The AI platform was no longer a guide through injury, but a companion in maintenance—a quiet presence helping him navigate complexity.

Standing at a window one evening, Marcus reflected on the long view. Healing was not about returning to a single version of himself, but about sustaining capacity across time. With adaptive intelligence supporting his awareness, the future felt less fragile. Recovery had become continuity, and growth felt possible not despite change, but because of it.

*Chapter 9*

# Neuroprotection, Relapse Prevention, and the AI Safety Net for the Healing Brain

Recovery from stroke or brain injury does not conclude when function stabilizes or when individuals return to daily routines. The healing brain remains vulnerable to relapse, secondary injury, and gradual decline influenced by stress, aging, vascular health, and lifestyle factors. Long-term success therefore depends not only on rehabilitation, but on neuroprotection—the active preservation of neural integrity and the prevention of future disruption. Artificial intelligence provides a powerful safety net in this phase by continuously monitoring risk signals, reinforcing protective behaviors, and intervening early when instability emerges.

Neuroprotection begins with understanding that the post-injury brain operates under different constraints. Neural networks that have reorganized to compensate for damage often function efficiently but with reduced redundancy. This means that stressors once tolerated may now produce disproportionate effects. AI systems track subtle changes in performance variability, reaction time drift, sleep disruption, and emotional volatility to identify early warning signs before symptoms escalate. This early detection enables preventative action rather than reactive treatment.

AI-driven relapse prevention reframes setbacks as signals rather than failures. Temporary declines in performance are common and often reversible when addressed promptly. Algorithms analyze deviations from baseline patterns to distinguish between normal variability and meaningful risk. When thresholds are crossed, AI systems recommend targeted interventions such as workload adjustments, cognitive rest, hydration, or medical review. This contextual interpretation reduces anxiety while preserving vigilance, helping individuals respond constructively rather than catastrophically.

Lifestyle factors play a decisive role in long-term brain stability. Sleep quality, cardiovascular health, nutrition, physical activity, and stress management all influence neuroplastic capacity and vulnerability. AI platforms integrate data from wearables and self-reports to correlate these factors with cognitive and emotional performance. Over time, the system identifies personalized risk profiles, highlighting which behaviors most strongly affect stability. Neuroprotection becomes individualized rather than generic, guided by evidence specific to the person rather than population averages. Medication adherence and medical follow-up also benefit from AI-supported monitoring. Post-stroke care often involves complex regimens that can be difficult to sustain. AI systems provide reminders, track adherence patterns, and flag deviations that may increase risk. When integrated with clinical oversight, these tools support continuity of care without replacing medical judgment. The safety net extends across domains, connecting daily behavior with long-term neurological health.

Stress is one of the most significant predictors of relapse and decline. Chronic stress disrupts neurotransmitter balance, impairs sleep, and weakens cognitive resilience. AI systems detect stress through physiological and behavioral markers, offering timely interventions such as breathing guidance, workload modification, or cognitive reframing exercises. By addressing stress proactively, AI protects the brain's adaptive capacity and reduces cumulative risk.

A critical component of neuroprotection is education. AI-generated insights help individuals understand their own patterns of vulnerability and resilience. This awareness empowers informed decision-making, enabling individuals to anticipate risk rather than react to crisis. Neuroprotection shifts from compliance to collaboration, with individuals actively participating in safeguarding their brain health. Ethical safeguards are essential in preventative monitoring. AI systems must balance vigilance with respect for autonomy, ensuring that recommendations remain supportive rather than intrusive. Transparency in how risk is assessed and how data is used builds trust, encouraging sustained engagement. Neuroprotection succeeds when individuals feel supported, not surveilled.

Ultimately, AI transforms long-term brain care from episodic intervention into continuous stewardship. By providing an intelligent safety net, AI reduces the likelihood of relapse, preserves hard-earned gains, and supports lifelong neural resilience. Recovery thus extends beyond healing into sustained protection, ensuring that the brain's capacity for adaptation remains intact over time.

### *Guardrails*

After returning to a full routine, Sophia believed the hardest part was behind her. She had regained confidence, resumed responsibilities, and settled into a rhythm that felt stable. Then subtle changes appeared—fatigue lingered longer, focus slipped under pressure, sleep became fragmented. Nothing dramatic enough to alarm others, but enough to unsettle her.

Sophia continued using an AI-supported monitoring system introduced during rehabilitation. The platform noticed what she hesitated to acknowledge: small deviations from her baseline. Reaction times slowed, emotional responses sharpened, recovery after stress lengthened. Instead of issuing warnings, the system offered context. Patterns suggested cumulative stress rather than neurological regression.

With this insight, Sophia adjusted. Workdays shortened slightly, sleep routines stabilized, stress management exercises reentered her schedule. The system tracked improvement, confirming that protective actions were working. Relief replaced fear as understanding took hold.

Weeks later, Sophia faced an unusually demanding period. The AI system anticipated risk, recommending pacing strategies before symptoms emerged. When she followed the guidance, stability held. The safety net worked not by preventing challenge, but by supporting resilience through it.

Sophia realized that recovery was not fragile—it was guarded. The AI platform did not promise certainty, but it provided guardrails that allowed confidence without complacency. She felt capable of navigating complexity, knowing early signals would not be ignored.

Standing in her kitchen one morning, clear-headed and calm, Sophia recognized that healing had matured into protection. The brain she had rebuilt was now supported by awareness, foresight, and intelligent care. Recovery had not ended; it had been safeguarded.

*Chapter 10*

# From Healing to Stewardship: Building a Lifelong AI-Guided Brain Health Strategy

The final stage of brain recovery is not an endpoint but a transition—from active healing to lifelong stewardship. Once foundational recovery is achieved and stability is established, the central question becomes how to protect, strengthen, and evolve brain health over decades rather than months. Stroke and brain injury often act as catalysts for deeper awareness of neurological vulnerability, but they also open the door to a more intentional relationship with cognitive well-being. Artificial intelligence supports this transition by shifting from rehabilitation guidance to long-term brain health strategy, transforming recovery into a durable, adaptive system of care.

Brain stewardship begins with the recognition that neuroplasticity does not expire. While the rate of change may slow, the brain continues to adapt in response to learning, stress, and environment throughout life. AI systems designed for long-term use monitor patterns across extended time horizons, identifying how daily behaviors influence neural resilience. Rather than focusing solely on performance metrics, stewardship models emphasize trend stability, recovery capacity, and adaptability under changing conditions. This broader lens reframes success as sustained capacity rather than peak output.

A key element of lifelong stewardship is anticipatory guidance. Instead of responding to symptoms after they arise, AI systems forecast risk by analyzing longitudinal data. Gradual shifts in attention span, emotional regulation, sleep architecture, or cognitive endurance can signal emerging vulnerability long before functional decline becomes visible. By detecting these early markers, AI enables preventative adjustments that preserve neural integrity. Stewardship thus prioritizes foresight over crisis management, reducing the likelihood of future disruption.

Personalization remains essential at this stage. Long-term brain health is influenced by unique genetic, environmental, and lifestyle factors that interact dynamically over time. AI systems refine personalized models continuously, updating recommendations as life circumstances evolve. Career changes, aging, health conditions, and stressors all reshape cognitive demands. Stewardship systems adapt accordingly, ensuring that guidance remains relevant rather than rigid. This flexibility prevents stagnation and supports ongoing alignment between brain capacity and life complexity.

Integration with physical health becomes increasingly important in lifelong brain care. Cardiovascular function, metabolic health, and inflammation significantly affect cognitive resilience. AI platforms synthesize data across these domains, highlighting connections between physical health trends and cognitive performance. By presenting these relationships clearly, AI empowers individuals to make informed choices that support whole-body, whole-brain stability. Stewardship becomes holistic, recognizing that the brain does not operate in isolation from the body it inhabits.

Emotional intelligence and meaning also play a role in long-term brain vitality. Chronic stress, unresolved trauma, and emotional disengagement erode neural resilience over time. AI systems that monitor emotional patterns help individuals recognize when psychological load exceeds adaptive capacity. By encouraging restorative practices and emotional regulation strategies, AI protects the neural foundations of cognition. Stewardship thus includes not only what the brain does, but how it experiences life.

Education is a cornerstone of sustainable stewardship. AI-guided insights transform abstract neuroscience into practical understanding, enabling individuals to interpret their own data with clarity. This literacy fosters autonomy, reducing dependence on external intervention. When individuals understand how their brain responds to choices and stressors, they become active custodians of their own neurological health rather than passive recipients of care.

Ethical stewardship demands transparency and choice. Lifelong AI systems must remain tools, not authorities. Individuals should retain control over goals, thresholds, and engagement levels. Successful stewardship frameworks prioritize collaboration, allowing users to accept, modify, or reject recommendations based on values and context. Trust sustains long-term engagement, and trust emerges only when agency is preserved.

Ultimately, lifelong AI-guided brain health represents a cultural shift in how recovery is understood. Healing does not conclude when symptoms resolve; it matures into intentional maintenance and growth. AI enables this evolution by providing continuity, insight, and adaptability across the lifespan. The brain, once injured, becomes not fragile but informed—supported by systems designed to honor its complexity and protect its future. Stewardship transforms recovery into a lasting relationship with resilience, learning, and purposeful living.

*The Custodian*

Ten years after her stroke, Eleanor no longer introduced herself as a survivor. The word felt too anchored to the past. She lived fully—worked part-time, traveled, volunteered—but she remained deeply aware of her brain in ways she had never been before. Not with fear, but with respect. Recovery had taught her that health was not something to assume; it was something to steward.

Eleanor still used an AI-guided brain health platform that had evolved with her over the years. It no longer asked her to complete exercises or track obvious deficits. Instead, it quietly observed patterns—how her focus shifted with sleep quality, how emotional stress affected decision-making, how periods of high engagement influenced fatigue. The system offered insights, not alarms. Suggestions, not commands.

When Eleanor noticed subtle mental fog during a particularly busy season, the AI system reflected what she suspected but hadn't fully acknowledged: cumulative stress was exceeding recovery capacity. Together, they adjusted. Commitments softened, rest increased, and clarity returned without drama. The safety net worked because it respected her autonomy, supporting decisions rather than dictating them. As Eleanor aged, the system adapted again. Cognitive endurance changed, priorities shifted, and the AI's guidance evolved accordingly. It helped her maintain engagement without overextension, curiosity without strain. Brain health became part of how she planned her life, not something she worried about in the background.

One afternoon, while mentoring a younger colleague recovering from injury, Eleanor realized how far she had come. She spoke not about fear or limitation, but about awareness and care. Recovery, she explained, had not ended—it had transformed into stewardship.

Walking home that evening, Eleanor felt grounded rather than vigilant. Her brain was not perfect, but it was protected, understood, and supported. Healing had become a lifelong partnership, not with technology alone, but with herself. The custodian of her own mind, she moved forward with confidence rooted in knowledge, not assumption.

# Epilogue

*The Healing Brain as a Living System*

This book has traced the journey of brain healing not as a single intervention, but as a living system—one that adapts, reorganizes, and strengthens across time when supported by the right conditions. Stroke and brain injury once represented an endpoint, a line drawn between ability and limitation. What has emerged instead is a new understanding: the brain is not a static organ that breaks and remains broken, but a dynamic network capable of recovery, compensation, and long-term resilience. Artificial intelligence does not create this capacity; it reveals it, supports it, and helps sustain it when human perception alone falls short.

AI's role in brain healing is not defined by novelty, speed, or technological sophistication, but by alignment. The most effective systems do not force change; they listen for it. They observe patterns of readiness, fatigue, emotion, and engagement, responding with calibrated guidance rather than rigid instruction. In doing so, AI mirrors the very principle it supports—plasticity. Recovery succeeds not because the brain is pushed relentlessly, but because effort is applied intelligently, in rhythm with biological reality. Throughout this book, one theme has remained constant: healing is contextual.

Physical recovery depends on cognitive clarity, emotional stability, identity coherence, and environmental support. AI's power lies in its ability to integrate these dimensions rather than treating them as separate domains. When movement, cognition, emotion, and behavior are addressed together, recovery becomes coherent rather than fragmented. The brain heals not in isolation, but in relationship—to tasks, people, meaning, and time.

Equally important is the shift from episodic care to continuity. Rehabilitation no longer ends when formal therapy concludes. With AI-supported systems, healing extends into daily life, adapting to changing demands and protecting against future instability. This continuity reframes recovery as stewardship, encouraging individuals to maintain and evolve brain health over the lifespan. What once required constant clinical oversight can now be guided by insight, awareness, and adaptive support.

Ethics remain central to this transformation. AI must serve human dignity, autonomy, and understanding. When systems are transparent, explainable, and collaborative, trust emerges naturally. The goal is not dependence on technology, but empowerment through insight. AI succeeds when individuals learn to recognize their own signals, using guidance as a tool rather than a crutch. Healing becomes participatory rather than prescriptive.

Perhaps the most profound outcome of AI-assisted brain healing is psychological. When recovery is understood as possible, adaptable, and ongoing, fear loses its grip. Individuals no longer define themselves by what was lost, but by what can still be built. This reframing restores agency, replacing uncertainty with informed choice. The brain becomes not a fragile liability, but a capable system deserving of care, respect, and investment.

As research and technology continue to evolve, new tools will emerge—more precise, more integrated, more powerful. Yet the foundation will remain unchanged. Healing depends on alignment between biology and behavior, between effort and timing, between support and autonomy. AI's role is to hold that alignment steady, adapting as life unfolds.

This book does not conclude with answers set in stone, but with principles meant to endure. Recovery is not linear. Progress is not permanent without care. Strength is not the absence of vulnerability, but the capacity to adapt when vulnerability appears. With AI as a partner—not a replacement—brain healing becomes not a miracle, but a methodical, humane process grounded in understanding. The future of neurorehabilitation is not defined by machines healing brains, but by humans learning how to support their own adaptability with intelligence, compassion, and foresight. In that future, recovery is not an exception. It is an expectation—guided, sustained, and lived.

### *The Last Appointment*

On the day of her final follow-up appointment, Laura arrived early and sat quietly in the waiting room. The space felt familiar, but distant, as if it belonged to an earlier version of herself. Years had passed since her stroke, years marked not by dramatic breakthroughs, but by steady, deliberate rebuilding. She no longer came here because she needed permission to move forward. She came to close a chapter.

Her neurologist reviewed the data collected over time—patterns of recovery, stability, adaptation. The AI-supported system that had guided her rehabilitation now showed something different: consistency. Variability still existed, but within healthy bounds. The brain she had rebuilt was not flawless, but it was resilient. The doctor smiled and said what Laura already knew. "You're not recovering anymore," he said. "You're maintaining."

Walking out of the clinic, Laura felt something unexpected—not relief, but clarity. The fear that once followed her everywhere was gone. In its place was awareness. She understood her limits, but she also understood her strength. The AI platform remained active, quietly monitoring trends, offering guidance when needed, but no longer commanding attention. It had become background knowledge, like a trusted map rather than a constant guide.

At home, Laura prepared dinner, moved through her evening routine, and reflected on how different life felt now. Recovery had not returned her to who she was before. It had shaped someone more attentive, more intentional, more patient. She noticed signs of fatigue earlier, respected rest without guilt, and approached challenge with curiosity rather than force.

Later that night, Laura reviewed a summary from her AI system—not warnings, not instructions, just reflection. Stability. Balance. Adaptation. She closed the app without ceremony. The data mattered, but it no longer defined her.

Standing by the window, watching the city lights settle into the evening, Laura realized that healing had quietly completed its transformation. What began as survival had become stewardship. What once required constant monitoring had become second nature. The brain she lived with was not something to fear or fix—it was something to care for.

There was no finish line to cross, no announcement to make. Life simply continued, supported by understanding rather than assumption. Laura turned off the light and went to bed, not thinking about recovery at all. And in that quiet normalcy, the journey found its truest ending.

www.ingramcontent.com/pod-product-compliance
Lightning Source LLC
LaVergne TN
LVHW022022200926
848481LV00007B/2499
*9798295627279*